INJURY REHABILITATION FOR SENIORS

Rebuild and Recover

Basil U

COPYRIGHT

TABLE OF CONTENTS

ABOUT THE BOOK

In a world where the aging population is rapidly increasing, the need for effective rehabilitation strategies tailored specifically for seniors has never been more critical. "Injury Rehabilitation for Seniors: Rebuild and Recover" is a comprehensive guide designed to address the unique challenges and needs of older adults on their journey to recovery after injury. This book serves not only as a practical resource but also as an inspiring roadmap for seniors and their caregivers, empowering them to reclaim their health and independence.

Understanding the Need for Specialized Rehabilitation

Aging brings about a variety of physiological changes that can complicate recovery from injury. Factors such as decreased bone density, loss of muscle mass, and reduced elasticity of connective tissues mean that seniors often face longer and more complex rehabilitation processes compared to younger individuals. Additionally, the presence of chronic conditions—such as arthritis, diabetes, or heart disease—can further complicate recovery efforts. Recognizing these challenges, this book provides targeted information and strategies tailored specifically for seniors, emphasizing the importance of personalized rehabilitation plans that consider the individual's unique health profile.

A Holistic Approach to Recovery

"Injury Rehabilitation for Seniors: Rebuild and Recover" goes beyond mere physical rehabilitation. The book adopts a holistic perspective, emphasizing the interconnectedness of physical, emotional, and mental well-being in the recovery process. Each chapter is infused with practical advice, personal anecdotes, and success stories that resonate with readers, illustrating the resilience of the human spirit. Readers will find that rehabilitation is not just about regaining strength and mobility; it's about fostering a sense of purpose, enhancing mental health, and cultivating supportive relationships.

Comprehensive Coverage of Rehabilitation Techniques

The book is structured to guide readers through every stage of the rehabilitation process. It begins with an exploration of how aging affects injury recovery and the necessity for customized care. Each chapter delves into specific types of injuries commonly faced by seniors, from hip fractures and joint replacements to falls and balance-related injuries. The authors provide evidence-based techniques for rehabilitation, including low-impact exercises, strength training, flexibility routines, and balance coordination practices.

In addition to physical therapy techniques, the book addresses the importance of pain management strategies, nutritional considerations for healing, and the mental and emotional aspects of recovery. With insights on managing setbacks, building confidence, and fostering social connections, the authors create a comprehensive framework that equips seniors with the tools necessary for a successful recovery journey.

Innovative Therapies and Advanced Treatments

"Injury Rehabilitation for Seniors: Rebuild and Recover" also highlights alternative therapies and advanced treatments that can complement traditional rehabilitation methods. Readers will learn about the benefits of hydrotherapy, electrical stimulation therapy, and mind-body practices like yoga and Tai Chi. These innovative approaches are not only effective in enhancing recovery but also contribute to a more enjoyable and fulfilling rehabilitation experience.

Practical Guidance for Home-Based Rehabilitation

Recognizing the importance of accessibility, the book emphasizes home-based rehabilitation techniques that seniors can incorporate into their daily routines. Practical advice on creating safe home environments, utilizing assistive devices, and accessing virtual therapy options ensure that readers have the resources they need to continue their rehabilitation journey independently.

Empowering Seniors and Caregivers

A significant focus of this book is to empower both seniors and their caregivers. By providing knowledge and strategies that are easy to understand and implement, "Injury Rehabilitation for Seniors: Rebuild and Recover" aims to build confidence and resilience. It encourages open communication between seniors and their healthcare providers, fostering collaborative efforts that enhance recovery outcomes.

Caregivers, too, will find invaluable insights on how to best support their loved ones during rehabilitation. The book addresses the emotional dynamics of caregiving and the importance of establishing a strong support system to ensure a smoother recovery process.

A Message of Hope and Resilience

Ultimately, "Injury Rehabilitation for Seniors: Rebuild and Recover" delivers a powerful message: recovery is a journey filled with opportunities for growth, resilience, and renewed independence. Through engaging storytelling and practical guidance, the authors inspire seniors to embrace the challenges of rehabilitation with determination and optimism.

This book is more than just a guide; it is a companion for seniors navigating the complexities of recovery. Whether recovering from a serious injury, managing chronic conditions, or simply seeking to maintain their health and independence, readers will find the support, knowledge, and inspiration they need to rebuild and recover successfully.

In conclusion, "Injury Rehabilitation for Seniors: Rebuild and Recover" is an essential resource for seniors, caregivers, and healthcare professionals alike. It recognizes the unique challenges faced by older adults in their recovery journeys and provides comprehensive, accessible strategies to promote healing, independence, and a fulfilling life. As readers turn the pages, they will discover not only how to heal their bodies but also how to cultivate a spirit of resilience and embrace the joys of life after injury.

INTRODUCTION

Aging brings about changes that many of us never expect. Muscles weaken, bones become more fragile, and even small injuries can feel like major setbacks. Yet, despite these challenges, the senior body remains remarkably resilient. With the right care and a well-structured rehabilitation program, seniors can rebuild strength, recover mobility, and regain confidence after injury. It's not just about healing; it's about reclaiming independence and continuing to live a life full of vitality.

Injury rehabilitation is particularly crucial for older adults, as it can prevent long-term disabilities that often stem from seemingly minor incidents. A fall, a twisted joint, or even overuse of muscles can lead to fractures, joint damage, or soft tissue injuries that may require months of healing. Without proper rehabilitation, these injuries can severely impact mobility, making everyday tasks difficult and reducing overall quality of life. But when seniors are guided through the right recovery plan, the potential to prevent these long-term issues is immense.

Consider this: a senior who suffers a hip fracture may fear they'll never walk unaided again. However, with a combination of targeted exercises, careful physical therapy, and emotional support, they can often return to full function. The same goes for common joint injuries, like those affecting the knees, shoulders, or ankles—rehabilitation can rebuild the strength needed to perform everyday activities and prevent future injuries.

At the heart of effective rehabilitation is setting realistic expectations. Recovery is not instantaneous; it takes time, patience, and commitment. The journey can be long, with milestones that may feel far apart. But knowing what to expect—and celebrating each small victory—can make all the difference. Whether it's regaining the ability to walk without assistance or simply being able to perform daily tasks independently, the rewards of rehabilitation are profound.

This book is a guide to rebuilding and recovering, not just for seniors, but for their families, caregivers, and loved ones. Through a combination of personal success stories, practical advice, and insights from medical professionals, we'll explore the many paths to recovery. The process may be challenging, but as we'll see through the pages ahead, the human body—especially in the later years—has an incredible capacity to heal and thrive with the right support.

CHAPTER 1

UNDERSTANDING SENIOR-SPECIFIC REHABILITATION NEEDS

Recovering from an injury is never a simple process, but for seniors, it presents unique challenges. The aging body responds differently to stress, and the pace of healing can vary greatly from that of a younger individual. To truly grasp how to support a senior through injury rehabilitation, we first need to understand the physiological changes that come with age, the need for personalized rehabilitation plans, and the additional complexity introduced by chronic conditions.

How Aging Affects Injury Recovery

Imagine a sprightly 30-year-old who twists their ankle while playing tennis. In just a few weeks, with rest and some ice, they're back on their feet and ready to go. Now, compare this to an 80-year-old who suffers a similar injury. The same twisted ankle may take months to heal, and without proper care, it could lead to complications that affect their overall mobility.

This difference in recovery isn't just about age but the changes in the body's tissues. As we age, our bones lose density—a condition commonly known as osteopenia, and in more severe cases, osteoporosis. Bones that were once strong and capable of absorbing impact become fragile, making fractures more likely and recovery slower. At the same time, muscle mass declines, a natural process called sarcopenia, which can lead to a loss of strength and endurance. Tissue elasticity, too, decreases with age, meaning that muscles, tendons, and ligaments are more prone to injury and take longer to heal.

For seniors, even simple tasks—like getting out of a chair or walking upstairs—can become hurdles in recovery. These changes make it critical to approach rehabilitation with patience and understanding. The body is still capable of incredible resilience, but it requires a gentler, more focused approach to regain its strength and function.

Customized Care: Tailoring Rehabilitation for Seniors

A one-size-fits-all approach does not work for senior rehabilitation. While younger individuals can often follow a standard recovery protocol, seniors need care that's tailored to their unique physical and medical needs. The first step in creating a customized plan is understanding the specific injury and its impact on daily life.

Let's take Mary's story, for instance. In her early 70s, she suffered a fall that resulted in a fractured hip. Her doctors recommended surgery, followed by rehabilitation. Initially, Mary was determined to recover quickly, but the pain was overwhelming, and she found it difficult to stick to the plan laid out for her. The exercises felt too strenuous, and her motivation waned. It wasn't until her physical therapist, Sarah, re-evaluated her program and adjusted it to suit her pace that Mary began to make real progress. Sarah incorporated gentle aquatic therapy, which allowed Mary to exercise in water without the strain on her joints. This simple adjustment changed everything, and soon Mary was regaining her strength and confidence.

Tailoring rehabilitation means taking the time to understand not only the injury but the senior's overall health, capabilities, and even their mindset. Some seniors may be eager to push themselves, while others, like Mary, may need a slower, more forgiving pace. Physical therapists, occupational therapists, and geriatric specialists play a critical role in creating these personalized programs. By focusing on exercises that are low-impact, safe, and targeted, they can help seniors achieve long-term recovery without risking re-injury.

Customized care also takes into account the senior's lifestyle. Are they living independently or with family? Do they have the support they need at home to continue their recovery when they're not in therapy? These questions help shape a rehabilitation plan that's not just effective in the clinic but also sustainable in everyday life.

Role of Chronic Conditions in Recovery

For many seniors, injury recovery is further complicated by chronic conditions like arthritis, diabetes, or heart disease. These conditions not only slow down the healing process but can also pose risks during rehabilitation.

Take arthritis, for example. For a senior dealing with joint pain, exercises that might be standard in a recovery plan could exacerbate their symptoms. Imagine trying to rehabilitate a knee injury when your joints are already inflamed and sore. It's a delicate balancing act. This is where an experienced therapist comes in, adapting exercises to be joint-friendly, incorporating stretches, and focusing on flexibility to ease the pain without sacrificing recovery.

Another challenge is diabetes, which can affect circulation and lead to slower wound healing. For seniors with diabetes, even a minor injury, like a cut or a bruise, requires careful attention. Poor circulation means the body's ability to deliver oxygen and nutrients to the injured site is impaired, and this delays recovery. Additionally, blood sugar levels need to be carefully monitored during physical activity to prevent spikes or crashes. In such cases, the rehabilitation process must be closely managed with a multidisciplinary approach, involving not just therapists but also the senior's primary care physician or endocrinologist.

Heart disease presents yet another hurdle. Seniors recovering from injury while managing heart conditions may find that their physical limitations extend beyond the injury itself. Cardiovascular health plays a huge role in the ability to participate in rehabilitation. Exercise is essential for recovery, but it must be balanced with heart health considerations. Low-intensity exercises, like walking, swimming, or stationary cycling, are often recommended to keep the heart healthy while rebuilding strength.

Let's not forget that many seniors are dealing with multiple chronic conditions at once. Take John, who at 76 is recovering from a shoulder injury. He also has diabetes and high blood pressure. His rehabilitation plan has to consider all of these factors. His physical therapist works closely with his doctor to ensure that his exercises are safe, that his blood sugar levels are stable, and that his heart rate stays within a safe range during his sessions. It's a team effort, and it requires constant communication between healthcare providers and the patient.

A Holistic Approach to Senior Rehabilitation

The process of rehabilitating seniors requires more than just physical recovery; it's about considering the whole person—their physical limitations, their emotional needs, and their long-term health. As we've seen, aging bodies recover differently from injuries. They require personalized care that takes into account not only the injury itself but the underlying health conditions that may slow or complicate the healing process.

By recognizing the unique needs of seniors in rehabilitation and taking a holistic approach to their care, we can help them regain their independence, strength, and quality of life. The road to recovery may be longer, and the challenges may be greater, but with the right support, seniors can rebuild and recover, often beyond what they thought possible.

CHAPTER 2

TYPES OF INJURIES COMMONLY FACED BY SENIORS

Injury is an inevitable part of life, but as we age, even a small misstep can lead to something more serious. For seniors, certain types of injuries are particularly common, especially those involving the joints, spine, and muscles. These injuries can make everyday tasks feel impossible, but recovery is not out of reach. With targeted rehabilitation and the right support, seniors can regain mobility and reclaim their independence. In this chapter, we'll explore some of the most common injuries faced by seniors and the rehabilitation approaches that help them recover.

Hip Fractures and Joint Replacement Recovery: Keys to Regaining Mobility

Few injuries strike fear into seniors like a hip fracture. It's one of the most common—and most serious—injuries in older adults. Hip fractures often occur after a fall, and the recovery process can be long and challenging. Many seniors worry that a fractured hip will rob them of their independence forever, but with proper rehabilitation, it doesn't have to.

Hip replacement surgeries, whether due to a fracture or arthritis, have become more routine in recent years. These surgeries offer a new lease on life, but the road to full mobility requires dedication. After surgery, the initial focus is on reducing pain and swelling, but once that's under control, it's all about movement.

The key to regaining mobility after a hip fracture or replacement is early rehabilitation. Simple tasks like getting out of bed, walking a few steps, and even sitting up can feel daunting. Physical therapy begins gently, with exercises designed to restore strength to the leg muscles, particularly those around the hip. Walking aids like crutches or walkers are often necessary in the early stages, but the goal is to transition to walking unaided over time.

For seniors like Barbara, who suffered a hip fracture at 79, recovery seemed overwhelming at first. But with the help of her physical therapist, she began to see progress. Her therapist started with small movements—lifting her leg while lying down, gently rotating her hip, and eventually, walking a few steps with a walker. Over time, those few steps turned into short walks around her home, and soon enough, Barbara was confident enough to venture outdoors. Her success story, like so many others, shows that with the right guidance, seniors can recover mobility even after serious injuries.

Falls and Balance-Related Injuries: The Role of Balance Exercises and Fall Prevention Strategies

Falls are a leading cause of injury in seniors, and they often result in fractures, sprains, or worse. The fear of falling can become a mental burden, making seniors hesitant to move freely and, paradoxically, increasing their risk of injury. When someone avoids movement, their muscles weaken, and their balance worsens, creating a vicious cycle.

To break this cycle, balance exercises and fall prevention strategies are critical components of rehabilitation. Simple balance exercises, such as standing on one leg or walking heel-to-toe, can make a world of difference. These exercises improve proprioception, the body's ability to sense its position in space, which is vital for avoiding falls.

Consider Tom, a 72-year-old who struggled with balance issues after a minor fall in his kitchen. His therapist introduced him to a balance training program, which began with standing on one foot while holding onto a chair for support. Over time, Tom graduated to more advanced exercises, like using a balance board. These exercises helped him not only recover from his fall but also gain the confidence to move around his home without fear.

In addition to exercises, fall prevention strategies are key. These include making the home safer by removing tripping hazards, ensuring adequate lighting, and using non-slip rugs. The combination of these practical adjustments and balance training reduces the risk of future falls.

Spine and Back Injuries: Approaches to Reducing Pain and Strengthening Core Muscles

Back pain is one of the most common complaints among seniors, and it often stems from spinal injuries or degenerative conditions like osteoporosis or arthritis. Whether it's a herniated disc, muscle strain, or chronic spinal condition, back pain can severely limit mobility and quality of life.

For seniors recovering from back injuries, reducing pain and strengthening core muscles is essential. The spine relies heavily on the surrounding muscles for support, so strengthening the core—specifically the abdominal and lower back muscles—plays a crucial role in alleviating pain and preventing future injuries.

Let's look at the case of Helen, a 68-year-old who experienced chronic lower back pain due to a herniated disc. Her rehabilitation focused on core-strengthening exercises like pelvic tilts, gentle yoga poses, and water-based activities. The buoyancy of the water took pressure off her spine while allowing her to engage her core. Over several months, Helen's pain lessened, and she was able to resume activities she had once thought impossible.

Stretching and posture correction are also important for spine health. Gentle stretches that target the back muscles, like cat-cow stretches or spinal twists, help alleviate tension. At the same time, correcting posture through awareness exercises can prevent further strain on the spine.

Shoulder, Knee, and Ankle Injuries: Specific Rehabilitation Exercises for These Common Joint Injuries

Shoulder, knee, and ankle injuries are especially prevalent among seniors, often due to wear and tear or accidents. These joints are essential for mobility, making their recovery vital for maintaining independence.

Shoulder injuries, such as rotator cuff tears or dislocations, can limit a person's ability to perform simple tasks like reaching for objects or dressing. Rehabilitation for shoulder injuries focuses on gentle range-of-motion exercises followed by strengthening the muscles that support the shoulder joint. Resistance bands are often used to help rebuild strength without putting undue stress on the joint.

Take the example of John, who dislocated his shoulder after slipping on wet pavement. His physical therapist started with passive movements, where the therapist moved John's arm for him, before gradually transitioning to active exercises like lifting small weights. Over time, John's shoulder regained its strength and flexibility, allowing him to return to his normal activities.

Knee injuries, whether from arthritis, meniscus tears, or ligament damage, can make walking and climbing stairs painful. Rehabilitation exercises for the knee often include leg lifts, step-ups, and squats, all designed to rebuild strength in the quadriceps and hamstrings. Strengthening these muscles provides better support for the knee joint, reducing pain and improving mobility.

Similarly, ankle injuries like sprains or fractures can take time to heal but are critical to address for maintaining balance and preventing falls. Rehabilitation for ankle injuries focuses on regaining range of motion through exercises like ankle circles, followed by strengthening exercises such as calf raises and resistance band work.

For seniors recovering from these joint injuries, consistency is key. Regularly performing rehabilitation exercises builds strength and flexibility, which are essential for preventing future injuries. The road to recovery may be long, but with patience and persistence, seniors can regain full function and independence.

Injury recovery for seniors may seem daunting, but understanding the nature of common injuries and the tailored rehabilitation exercises for each is the first step toward regaining strength and mobility. With the right approach, seniors can overcome these challenges and continue living active, fulfilling lives.

CHAPTER 3

STEP-BY-STEP GUIDE TO STARTING A REHABILITATION PROGRAM

Beginning a rehabilitation program after an injury can feel overwhelming, especially for seniors who may be unsure of where to start. But the process doesn't have to be intimidating. With the right guidance, the journey toward recovery becomes much clearer. In this chapter, we'll walk through the essential steps of getting started with rehabilitation, from receiving a proper diagnosis to creating a personalized plan and choosing the right professionals to help you on your path to healing.

Getting Diagnosed and Setting Goals: The First Steps After Injury

The first step toward recovery is understanding the extent of the injury. A proper diagnosis is crucial because it provides a roadmap for rehabilitation. Without it, you're essentially walking in the dark, unsure of how to approach healing or what to expect.

Imagine you've sprained your ankle during a fall. The pain is sharp, and the swelling makes it difficult to walk. You might think it'll heal on its own with rest, but without seeing a doctor, you don't know if there's more severe damage beneath the surface—such as a torn ligament. Seeking a professional diagnosis ensures that the injury is fully understood and that the appropriate treatment plan can be created.

Once you have a diagnosis, the next step is setting realistic goals for recovery. Goal-setting is an important part of rehabilitation because it gives you something to strive for. Start small and build your way up. For example, if you've fractured your hip, your initial goal might be to walk a few steps with a walker. Over time, that goal might evolve into walking unaided or climbing stairs.

Take the case of James, a 78-year-old who broke his hip in a fall. When he first began his rehabilitation, his goal was simply to sit up in bed without pain. As the weeks passed and his therapy progressed, his goals expanded. Soon, he was walking short distances with a cane, and eventually, he could walk around his neighborhood without assistance. Setting these small, attainable goals kept James motivated and gave him a clear sense of progress.

Choosing the Right Rehabilitation Professionals: Physical Therapists, Occupational Therapists, and Geriatric Specialists

The next step in starting a rehabilitation program is finding the right team of professionals to guide your recovery. Each type of specialist brings unique expertise to the table, and understanding their roles can help you choose the right support.

- Physical Therapists (PTs): Physical therapists are often the first professional's seniors work with after an injury. They focus on restoring movement, improving strength, and reducing pain through exercises and stretches. Whether you're recovering from a fracture, surgery, or a soft tissue injury, a PT is essential in helping you regain mobility.

- Occupational Therapists (OTs): Occupational therapists work on helping you return to everyday activities, such as dressing, bathing, and cooking. They often come into play when an injury affects your ability to perform these tasks independently. OTs can teach you ways to adapt your routine to accommodate your injury while you heal.

- Geriatric Specialists: These professionals specialize in working with seniors and are particularly helpful when managing the unique challenges of aging bodies. They understand how chronic conditions like arthritis or diabetes interact with injury recovery and can help tailor rehabilitation to fit your specific needs.

The story of Alice, a 74-year-old recovering from a knee replacement, highlights the importance of having the right professionals. Alice worked with a PT to strengthen her leg muscles and regain her ability to walk, but she also saw an OT who helped her adjust her home environment. Together, they ensured Alice could safely navigate her kitchen and bathroom while recovering. The collaborative efforts of both professionals played a huge role in Alice's successful rehabilitation.

Designing a Personalized Rehabilitation Plan: Key Components for Effective Recovery

Once you've chosen your rehabilitation team, the next step is designing a personalized plan tailored to your injury, abilities, and recovery goals. A good rehabilitation plan typically involves three core components: stretching, strengthening, and mobility exercises. Each part plays a crucial role in regaining your independence and preventing further injury.

- Stretching: Flexibility decreases with age, and injury can exacerbate stiffness in the muscles and joints. Stretching is an essential part of rehabilitation because it helps improve range of motion, making movement easier and less painful. For example, gentle hamstring stretches can help seniors recovering from hip or knee injuries regain the ability to walk comfortably.

- Strengthening: Strength is often lost during injury recovery, particularly in seniors who may already be dealing with muscle atrophy. Strengthening exercises focus on rebuilding muscle mass to support injured joints and bones. After a shoulder injury, for instance, exercises that target the rotator cuff muscles can help stabilize the shoulder and prevent re-injury.

- Mobility: Regaining the ability to move freely is a primary goal of rehabilitation. Mobility exercises, such as walking, climbing stairs, or even practicing standing from a seated position, help seniors return to their daily routines. These exercises are gradual and progress as the injury heals.

For James, whose story we explored earlier, his rehabilitation plan was carefully tailored to his needs. His therapist began with gentle stretching exercises to loosen his hip joint. As he improved, strengthening exercises like leg lifts were added. Finally, mobility work helped James transition from walking with a walker to using a cane, and eventually, to walking unaided.

Incorporating Assistive Devices: When and How to Use Canes, Walkers, or Wheelchairs During Rehab

During the rehabilitation process, assistive devices like canes, walkers, or wheelchairs can be invaluable tools. These devices provide support while seniors regain strength and mobility, helping prevent falls or re-injury. The key is knowing when and how to use them properly.

Assistive devices are often introduced early in rehabilitation when the body is still healing and not strong enough to bear weight independently. Canes, for example, can help relieve pressure on an injured leg or hip, while walkers offer more stability for those recovering from serious injuries like fractures.

It's important to remember that assistive devices should be viewed as temporary supports rather than permanent solutions. As rehabilitation progresses, the goal is to gradually reduce reliance on these tools. Barbara, who had fractured her hip, began her recovery using a walker. Over time, as her strength and balance improved, she transitioned to a cane and eventually no longer needed any support.

When using assistive devices, proper technique is essential. For example, when using a cane, it should be held in the hand opposite the injured leg to provide optimal support. Similarly, walkers should be used with slow, deliberate steps to ensure stability. Your physical therapist will guide you on how to use these devices correctly.

Starting a rehabilitation program after an injury can seem daunting, but it's a process built on small steps. With a proper diagnosis, the right professionals, and a personalized plan, recovery becomes much more achievable. Incorporating assistive devices as needed provides support along the way, ensuring that seniors can rebuild strength, regain mobility, and get back to their everyday lives.

CHAPTER 4

PHYSICAL THERAPY TECHNIQUES FOR SENIOR INJURY

REHABILITATION

Rehabilitation through physical therapy plays a vital role in helping seniors recover from injuries. By focusing on exercises that enhance mobility, strength, flexibility, and balance, physical therapy not only addresses the injury itself but also works to prevent future complications. In this chapter, we'll explore some of the most effective physical therapy techniques tailored to seniors, breaking down low-impact exercises, strengthening programs, flexibility routines, and balance practices that can make a significant difference in the recovery journey.

Low-Impact Exercises for Joint Health: Swimming, Cycling, and Walking

For seniors recovering from injuries, joint health is often a major concern. As we age, our joints become less resilient, and the wrong type of exercise can lead to pain or further injury. This is why low-impact exercises are highly recommended—they offer the benefits of movement and strength-building without placing undue stress on the joints.

- Swimming: One of the best low-impact exercises for seniors is swimming. Water provides natural resistance, which helps strengthen muscles while reducing the strain on joints. In fact, many rehabilitation programs include aquatic therapy sessions, where seniors perform exercises in a pool. The buoyancy of the water makes it easier to move, even for those with conditions like arthritis. Linda, a 76-year-old recovering from knee surgery, found that swimming was her lifeline. The water supported her body, making it possible to move her legs and build strength without pain.

- Cycling: Another excellent low-impact option is cycling. Stationary bikes are commonly used in physical therapy because they allow seniors to build leg strength and improve cardiovascular health without the jarring motion that comes with high-impact activities like running. For individuals recovering from hip or knee injuries, cycling helps restore range of motion while strengthening the muscles around the joints.

- Walking: Walking remains one of the simplest and most accessible low-impact exercises for seniors. It helps maintain joint health, strengthens muscles, and promotes cardiovascular fitness. After an injury, therapists often start with short, gentle walks, gradually increasing the distance and intensity as the senior's mobility improves. Bob, who suffered a back injury, started with walking around his house with the aid of a cane. Over time, he progressed to walking in his garden, and eventually, he was able to take daily strolls around his neighborhood, strengthening his back and legs.

Strengthening Programs for Seniors: Resistance Training and Bodyweight Exercises

Strengthening exercises are a cornerstone of injury rehabilitation for seniors. As we age, we naturally lose muscle mass, which can slow recovery and increase the risk of further injury. Resistance training and bodyweight exercises are key to rebuilding muscle strength, providing the foundation needed to support joints and improve overall mobility.

- Resistance Training: Using resistance bands or light weights, seniors can safely strengthen muscles without overloading the body. These exercises target key muscle groups, particularly those that support injured joints. For instance, after a shoulder injury, resistance band exercises that focus on the rotator cuff muscles can help rebuild strength and stabilize the joint. Similarly, leg-strengthening exercises using ankle weights are often prescribed for individuals recovering from hip or knee injuries. Mildred, an 80-year-old recovering from a hip fracture, found that resistance band exercises improved her leg strength and gave her the confidence to walk again.

- Bodyweight Exercises: These exercises use the weight of the body itself to build muscle and are often a key component of senior rehabilitation programs. Simple movements like squats, lunges, or modified push-ups can be done under the supervision of a therapist. These exercises help rebuild core strength, which is crucial for maintaining balance and preventing future falls. After a spine injury, John, aged 72, incorporated bodyweight exercises into his rehabilitation routine.

By strengthening his core, he not only reduced his back pain but also improved his posture and overall mobility.

Flexibility and Stretching Routines: Maintaining Range of Motion in Aging Joints

Flexibility often diminishes as we age, and this can be further exacerbated by injuries. Maintaining or improving flexibility is essential for seniors, particularly during rehabilitation, as it helps prevent stiffness, enhances range of motion, and reduces the risk of re-injury.

- Stretching Routines: Stretching is a simple yet powerful tool for injury recovery. Regular stretching improves circulation to injured areas and promotes healing by keeping muscles and joints supple. Common stretches used in senior rehabilitation include hamstring stretches, shoulder stretches, and gentle neck stretches. These can be done daily or as part of a broader therapy routine. Margaret, who struggled with shoulder pain after a fall, found that daily stretching routines helped her regain full range of motion in her shoulder and significantly reduced her discomfort.

- Maintaining Range of Motion: To keep aging joints healthy, it's essential to maintain a full range of motion. Stretching exercises like the seated leg extension (for the knees) or ankle circles (for ankle flexibility) are simple but effective. They can often be performed at home with minimal equipment, making them ideal for seniors who want to continue their rehabilitation outside of therapy sessions.

Balance and Coordination Exercises: Preventing Future Falls and Improving Proprioception

One of the most significant concerns for seniors is the risk of falling, especially after an injury. Falls can lead to serious complications, including fractures and head injuries. Incorporating balance and coordination exercises into a rehabilitation program can help prevent future falls by improving proprioception (the body's sense of its position in space) and strengthening stabilizing muscles.

- Balance Exercises: Balance exercises, such as standing on one leg or walking in a straight line, are often included in rehabilitation programs for seniors. These exercises train the body to maintain stability, even in challenging positions. For those recovering from hip or ankle injuries, balance exercises are particularly beneficial. For example, after an ankle sprain, Anna, aged 70, worked with her therapist to practice standing on one foot for increasing amounts of time. This improved her balance and confidence when walking.
- Coordination Drills: Simple coordination drills, like moving the feet in specific patterns or performing exercises that require the coordination of arms and legs simultaneously, help seniors develop better control over their movements. These

drills can also be fun and engaging, helping to make rehabilitation feel less like a chore. David, an 82-year-old recovering from a stroke, found that coordination exercises improved his mobility and made it easier for him to navigate his home safely.

Physical therapy techniques are central to injury rehabilitation for seniors, offering a comprehensive approach to recovery that includes low-impact exercises for joint health, strength-building routines, flexibility work, and balance training. By focusing on these areas, seniors can not only heal from their injuries but also build a stronger, more resilient body that's better equipped to handle the challenges of aging. Through the stories of people like Linda, Bob, Mildred, John, Margaret, Anna, and David, we see how these techniques can truly transform lives—helping seniors regain their independence, reduce pain, and prevent future injuries.

CHAPTER 5

MANAGING PAIN DURING RECOVERY

Pain is a natural part of the recovery process, especially for seniors healing from injuries. It's important to address this pain effectively to ensure that rehabilitation progresses smoothly, without unnecessary discomfort slowing things down. Pain management, however, isn't one-size-fits-all. There are many different approaches to dealing with pain, ranging from non-pharmacological methods like massage therapy and acupuncture to medications that provide relief. In this chapter, we will explore the various options available to seniors, looking at both conventional and holistic methods, and discussing how to manage pain safely and effectively during the rehabilitation process.

Non-Pharmacological Pain Management: Massage Therapy, Heat/Cold Applications, and Acupuncture

For seniors, non-pharmacological methods of pain relief can be an attractive option, particularly for those looking to avoid the risks associated with long-term medication use. These methods can often complement physical therapy by reducing pain and inflammation, improving circulation, and promoting relaxation, all of which contribute to the healing process.

- Massage Therapy: Massage therapy is a powerful tool for reducing pain, particularly in muscles and soft tissue. After an injury, muscles often become tight and sore due to inactivity or compensatory movements. Massage helps release this tension, improving blood flow to the injured area and promoting relaxation. Additionally, massage can reduce the pain of conditions like arthritis or sciatica, common issues that seniors often face during rehabilitation. For instance, after a shoulder injury, Paul, aged 75, found relief through weekly massage therapy sessions. The massages eased the muscle stiffness around his shoulder, allowing him to move more freely and participate fully in his physical therapy exercises.

- Heat and Cold Applications: Heat and cold therapy are simple yet highly effective methods for managing pain. Cold packs are often used immediately after an injury to reduce swelling and numb the area, providing short-term pain relief. On the other hand, heat therapy can be useful for relaxing tight muscles, easing chronic pain, and improving circulation. Seniors recovering from injuries like sprains, fractures, or joint replacements often alternate between heat and cold applications. Susan, who underwent knee replacement surgery at age 82, found that applying a cold pack after physical therapy sessions helped reduce the swelling in her knee, while heat therapy at night helped soothe her aching muscles and prepare her for a good night's sleep.

- Acupuncture: Acupuncture, an ancient practice rooted in traditional Chinese medicine, is another non-pharmacological method that has gained popularity for pain management. Tiny needles are inserted into specific points on the body, stimulating nerves, muscles, and connective tissue. For some seniors, acupuncture can reduce pain and inflammation, improve mobility, and promote overall well-being. After struggling with chronic back pain for years, Sarah, aged 80, turned to acupuncture during her rehabilitation. To her surprise, regular acupuncture sessions significantly reduced her pain levels and helped her regain mobility in her spine.

Medications and Senior Rehabilitation: Painkillers, Anti-Inflammatories, and Their Safe Usage

While non-pharmacological treatments are effective for many, there are times when medication is necessary to manage pain during recovery. Seniors, however, must approach medication with care. As the body ages, it becomes more sensitive to certain medications, and the risk of side effects increases. That's why it's important to use painkillers and anti-inflammatories judiciously and under the guidance of a healthcare professional.

- Painkillers: Common pain relievers, such as acetaminophen (Tylenol) or non-steroidal anti-inflammatory drugs (NSAIDs) like ibuprofen, are frequently prescribed to seniors recovering from injuries. These medications can help manage moderate pain and reduce inflammation, making it easier to engage in physical therapy and daily activities. However, seniors must be cautious about dosage and duration. Long-term use of NSAIDs, for example, can lead to gastrointestinal issues, kidney problems, or even increased blood pressure. Mary, aged 78, who was recovering from a hip fracture, found that a low-dose painkiller helped her get through her physical therapy sessions, but she worked closely with her doctor to gradually reduce the dosage as her recovery progressed.

- Anti-Inflammatories: Inflammation is a common response to injury, and while it's part of the body's healing process, too much inflammation can lead to pain and swelling. Anti-inflammatory medications, both over-the-counter and prescription, can reduce this swelling and make it easier to move and heal. After experiencing severe joint inflammation from a fall, Henry, aged 85, was prescribed a short course of anti-inflammatories. His doctor monitored him closely, ensuring that the medication was effective without causing side effects. Within weeks, his swelling decreased, allowing him to move more freely and progress in his rehabilitation.

- Safe Medication Practices for Seniors: Medication safety is crucial for seniors, as aging bodies process drugs differently than younger ones. It's important to follow dosage instructions carefully, avoid mixing medications without consulting a doctor, and be aware of any potential side effects. For those on multiple medications due to chronic conditions, working with a healthcare provider to manage drug interactions is essential. A personalized approach, balancing the benefits of medication with the risks, is key to managing pain effectively during rehabilitation.

Holistic Approaches: Mindfulness, Meditation, and Stress Management to Support Healing

Beyond physical treatments and medications, the mind plays a powerful role in the body's recovery process. Holistic approaches to pain management, such as mindfulness and meditation, offer seniors tools to manage their pain on a deeper level. These methods help not only with the physical aspect of recovery but also with the emotional and mental challenges that often accompany injury rehabilitation.

- Mindfulness and Meditation: Mindfulness involves paying attention to the present moment, focusing on the body's sensations without judgment. For seniors recovering from injuries, mindfulness practices can help reduce the perception of pain, decrease anxiety, and improve overall well-being. Meditation, often combined with mindfulness, teaches individuals to relax, breathe deeply, and focus their thoughts. By learning to shift attention away from the pain and onto something calming, seniors can experience a reduction in pain intensity. For example, Doris, aged 79, began practicing mindfulness meditation after a car accident left her with chronic neck pain. She found that daily meditation sessions helped her stay calm, focus on her recovery, and manage her pain without needing higher doses of medication.
- Stress Management: Injuries often lead to increased stress, which can worsen the perception of pain. Seniors may worry about their independence, their ability to return to normal activities, or the impact their injury will have on loved ones.

Managing stress is crucial for effective pain management. Techniques such as deep breathing, progressive muscle relaxation, or even listening to soothing music can help reduce tension in the body and make pain more manageable. For seniors like Tom, who struggled with stress after a knee injury, simple breathing exercises became a regular part of his recovery routine. Over time, he noticed not only a decrease in his stress levels but also an improvement in his ability to cope with pain.

Pain is a natural companion to injury, but it doesn't have to derail recovery. By combining non-pharmacological approaches like massage therapy, heat/cold applications, and acupuncture with safe use of medications and holistic techniques such as mindfulness and stress management, seniors can navigate the pain of rehabilitation in a balanced and effective way. Through the experiences of people like Paul, Susan, Sarah, Mary, Henry, Doris, and Tom, we see how different pain management strategies can be personalized to meet individual needs—leading not only to reduced pain but also to a smoother, more successful recovery journey.

CHAPTER 6

NUTRITION FOR HEALING AND RECOVERY

Nutrition plays a critical role in the healing process, especially for seniors recovering from injury. Just as physical therapy strengthens muscles and improves mobility, the right nutrients fuel the body, allowing it to rebuild and repair itself. As we age, however, the body's nutritional needs change, making it even more important to focus on the right foods that can support recovery. In this chapter, we will explore the essential nutrients for bone health, how to incorporate anti-inflammatory foods into the diet, and the vital role hydration plays in keeping the body on the path to healing.

Bone Health and Healing: Nutrients Like Calcium, Vitamin D, and Protein for Recovery

One of the most important aspects of recovery for seniors is ensuring the body has the nutrients it needs to strengthen bones and support tissue repair. Injuries like fractures, joint replacements, or soft tissue damage often require the body to build new bone and repair damaged tissues, and this process depends heavily on calcium, vitamin D, and protein.

- Calcium: Calcium is the building block of strong bones. For seniors, especially those recovering from fractures or undergoing joint replacement surgeries, maintaining an adequate intake of calcium is crucial. It helps ensure that bones remain strong and resilient, preventing further fractures or injuries. Foods rich in calcium, like dairy products, leafy greens, and fortified plant-based milks, are excellent sources. Take Linda, for example, a 76-year-old recovering from a hip fracture. Her doctor emphasized the importance of including calcium-rich foods in her diet, and she added more yogurt, almonds, and kale to her meals. This not only helped her regain strength but also improved her overall bone health as she aged.

- Vitamin D: While calcium is essential for bone strength, it cannot be absorbed properly without vitamin D. This vitamin plays a crucial role in bone metabolism, helping the body absorb calcium from the diet and maintain healthy bone tissue. Seniors often experience a deficiency in vitamin D, especially if they spend limited time outdoors. To improve recovery, seniors can incorporate vitamin D-rich foods such as fatty fish (like salmon), fortified cereals, and egg yolks. Some, like Michael, aged 80, found that a vitamin D supplement recommended by his doctor gave his bones the support they needed during his recovery from a shoulder injury.

- Protein: While calcium and vitamin D are key to bone health, protein is the foundation for repairing and building muscle tissue. After an injury, the body requires more protein than usual to rebuild damaged tissues, strengthen muscles, and maintain muscle mass. Seniors may struggle with protein intake, but focusing on lean meats, fish, beans, nuts, and legumes can help ensure adequate consumption. Joan, a 78-year-old woman recovering from knee surgery, increased her intake of fish and beans as part of her rehabilitation plan. Her physical therapist noted that her muscle strength improved rapidly, which helped her regain mobility sooner than expected.

Anti-Inflammatory Foods: Promoting Healing and Reducing Inflammation with the Right Diet

Inflammation is the body's natural response to injury, but when it becomes chronic or excessive, it can slow down the healing process. For seniors, managing inflammation through diet is an important part of rehabilitation. Certain foods contain natural anti-inflammatory properties that can help reduce swelling, ease discomfort, and promote faster healing.

- Omega-3 Fatty Acids: Omega-3 fatty acids, found in fish like salmon, sardines, and mackerel, as well as in flaxseeds and walnuts, have been shown to reduce inflammation in the body. These healthy fats support the immune system and help regulate the inflammatory response, which is especially beneficial for seniors recovering from joint injuries or fractures. Janet, aged 81, who was dealing with chronic inflammation in her joints due to arthritis, made the shift to include more omega-3-rich foods in her diet. She noticed that not only did her joint pain ease, but her recovery from a recent ankle injury was much smoother as well.

- Fruits and Vegetables: Brightly colored fruits and vegetables, such as berries, oranges, leafy greens, and bell peppers, are packed with antioxidants and vitamins that help reduce inflammation. These foods contain compounds like vitamin C, which supports collagen production—a key element in tissue repair. John, recovering from spinal surgery at age 85, made a conscious effort to include a variety of colorful fruits and vegetables in his diet, often blending berries into his morning smoothie. This helped him keep inflammation at bay while providing his body with the vitamins needed for a full recovery.

- Turmeric and Ginger: Both turmeric and ginger have long been known for their anti-inflammatory properties. Turmeric, in particular, contains curcumin, a compound that has been shown to reduce inflammation and support joint health. Ginger, commonly used in teas or added to meals, also has anti-inflammatory effects and can help ease pain and swelling. Seniors like Paul, who had suffered a back injury, added turmeric supplements to his recovery regimen and regularly drank ginger tea. He found that his pain levels were more manageable, and his physical therapist noted improvements in his range of motion.

Hydration and Its Role in Recovery: Keeping Muscles and Tissues Healthy

Staying hydrated may seem like an obvious part of health, but its role in injury recovery is often underestimated. Water is essential for nearly every function in the body, including circulation, muscle function, and tissue repair. For seniors, staying properly hydrated is critical to maintaining flexibility, preventing muscle cramps, and ensuring that nutrients are efficiently delivered to injured areas.

- Maintaining Muscle Health: Muscles are made up of about 75% water, so staying hydrated helps them function properly, especially during rehabilitation exercises. When the body is dehydrated, muscles become more prone to cramping and fatigue, which can hinder progress in physical therapy. Susan, 79, recovering from a hip fracture, made it a point to drink plenty of water before and after her rehabilitation sessions. She found that she experienced fewer muscle cramps and was able to perform her exercises with greater ease.

- Supporting Tissue Repair: Hydration also plays a vital role in keeping tissues healthy and aiding in the repair of damaged cells. Water helps maintain the elasticity of tissues, which is crucial when the body is healing from an injury. For seniors who may already have reduced tissue elasticity due to aging, proper hydration ensures that tissues remain pliable and resilient. Tom, who was recovering from shoulder surgery at age 82, noticed that his flexibility improved significantly when he focused on drinking more water throughout the day.

- Combatting Dehydration Risks in Seniors: Dehydration is a common risk for seniors, as the body's sense of thirst diminishes with age. This can lead to reduced muscle function, delayed recovery, and an increased risk of injury. Seniors need to be mindful of their hydration habits, drinking water regularly even if they don't feel thirsty. Incorporating hydrating foods like cucumbers, watermelon, and citrus fruits can also help. Mary, 84, learned the hard way after suffering dehydration during her recovery from a fall. Once her doctor emphasized the importance of hydration, she made it a habit to drink water throughout the day and found her energy levels and healing improved rapidly.

Nutrition is an essential, often overlooked part of the recovery process for seniors. By focusing on bone health with calcium, vitamin D, and protein, reducing inflammation through anti-inflammatory foods, and maintaining proper hydration, seniors can give their bodies the tools they need to heal effectively. Whether it's Linda adding more calcium to her meals, John embracing antioxidant-rich fruits, or Susan ensuring she drinks enough water, each of these stories shows that nutrition can make a powerful difference in the journey of rebuilding and recovering. The right dietary choices are not only about improving physical recovery but also about setting the foundation for long-term health and strength.

CHAPTER 7

MENTAL AND EMOTIONAL ASPECTS OF RECOVERY

Recovering from an injury isn't just a physical journey; it's also a mental and emotional one. For seniors, the road to recovery can feel longer and more challenging, particularly when progress is slow or setbacks occur. Mental resilience, emotional support, and a positive outlook can be just as critical to rehabilitation as physical therapy or medication. In this chapter, we'll explore how to cope with setbacks, conquer fears about re-injury, and cultivate strong support systems to stay motivated throughout the healing process.

Coping with Setbacks: How to Stay Motivated When Progress Feels Slow

Recovery is rarely linear. Seniors often face ups and downs, with good days followed by frustrating plateaus. When progress stalls or an unexpected complication arises, it's easy to feel discouraged. Understanding that setbacks are a natural part of the recovery process can help mitigate frustration and keep the focus on the bigger picture.

Take the story of Evelyn, for example, a 74-year-old woman who was making steady progress after a hip replacement surgery. Just as she started feeling stronger and more mobile, a bout of muscle stiffness set her back, requiring her to slow down her physical therapy sessions. Evelyn felt frustrated at first, doubting whether she would ever regain her full strength. But with the support of her physical therapist and family, she learned to celebrate the small victories—like walking a few extra steps each day or experiencing less pain. Her therapist reminded her that healing is like climbing a mountain: the ascent is gradual, but every step forward brings you closer to the summit.

To stay motivated during slow phases of recovery, it's important to break down long-term goals into smaller, achievable milestones. This allows you to recognize progress in smaller doses, whether it's being able to perform a new stretch, lift a little more weight, or walk for a longer period. Progress, no matter how incremental, is still progress. Visualization techniques can also be helpful. Picturing yourself living pain-free or moving comfortably again can keep the focus on where you're heading, rather than the challenges of the present moment.

Overcoming Anxiety and Fear of Re-Injury: Building Confidence Post-Injury

Injury can leave seniors feeling vulnerable and anxious about reinjury. It's common to feel hesitant or fearful about resuming normal activities, especially if the injury was caused by something as unpredictable as a fall. This fear can lead to avoidance, which can ultimately slow down recovery and lead to further issues like muscle weakness or stiffness.

Consider the experience of Harold, who was 80 when he fractured his wrist after slipping on a wet floor. After months of rehabilitation, Harold regained most of his mobility but found himself avoiding simple activities like gardening or even walking his dog for fear of falling again. He constantly replayed the fall in his mind, imagining how it could happen again in a different setting. His confidence was shaken, making it difficult to fully embrace his recovery.

Building confidence post-injury is a gradual process. It begins with reestablishing trust in your body's ability to heal and protect itself. Working closely with a physical therapist can help in this regard. Therapists often teach seniors specific exercises to strengthen the muscles around the injured area, ensuring that they have the stability and balance needed to avoid reinjury. Gradually reintroducing activities in a controlled and supervised environment can also help seniors regain confidence. Harold, for instance, started taking short walks with his physical therapist by his side, until he was comfortable walking on his own again.

Mindfulness techniques, like deep breathing and meditation, can also help manage anxiety. These practices allow seniors to stay present, rather than dwelling on past injuries or worrying about the future. Over time, Harold learned to replace his fear of falling with an appreciation for the progress he had made, building his confidence one step at a time.

Support Systems and Social Connections: The Role of Family, Friends, and Caregivers in Rehabilitation

The mental and emotional aspects of recovery are made easier with strong support systems. Rehabilitation is challenging, but having family, friends, and caregivers on your side can provide the encouragement needed to stay on track. Seniors who have a reliable network of people cheering them on tend to be more motivated and optimistic about their recovery.

Take Margaret's story, for instance. Margaret, 79, broke her ankle after a fall and had to spend several weeks in a rehabilitation center. During her stay, her daughter visited every day, helping with exercises and bringing her favorite meals to lift her spirits. Her friends from church sent her notes of encouragement and made plans to visit as soon as she returned home. Knowing she had a community that cared about her made all the difference in Margaret's recovery. She didn't feel isolated or forgotten. Instead, she felt supported, which kept her motivated to push through even the toughest therapy sessions.

Caregivers—whether family members or professional aides—also play a critical role in rehabilitation. They can assist with daily activities, remind seniors to perform their exercises, and ensure they're adhering to their rehabilitation plan. Caregivers often act as emotional anchors, helping seniors manage the frustration and emotional toll that comes with recovery.

One of the key elements of successful rehabilitation is communication. Seniors recovering from injuries should feel comfortable talking openly with their family, friends, and caregivers about their physical and emotional struggles. This dialogue allows for realistic expectations and emotional support when things don't go as planned. Caregivers, in particular, should be encouraged to offer not just physical assistance but emotional encouragement as well. A simple word of praise or reassurance can go a long way in boosting morale.

For those who may not have close family or friends nearby, rehabilitation groups or community support programs can fill that gap. Many seniors benefit from joining rehabilitation classes or support groups where they can connect with others who are going through similar experiences. In these settings, the shared understanding of injury and recovery fosters camaraderie and mutual support, reducing feelings of loneliness or isolation.

The Power of Positivity in Recovery

There's a saying: "Healing is an attitude." While physical therapy and proper medical care are essential, maintaining a positive attitude throughout the recovery process can make a world of difference. Positivity doesn't mean ignoring the hard parts of recovery; it means focusing on what's possible, even in the face of setbacks. Research has shown that seniors who maintain a positive outlook tend to experience faster recovery times and better overall outcomes.

Of course, staying positive isn't always easy, especially when progress feels slow or pain lingers. This is where support systems, coping strategies, and confidence-building techniques come into play. The goal is not to avoid difficult emotions but to navigate them with the understanding that recovery is a journey, not a race.

Mental and emotional resilience is just as important as physical strength in the recovery process. By learning to cope with setbacks, overcoming fears of reinjury, and leaning on a supportive network of family, friends, and caregivers, seniors can approach their rehabilitation with confidence and determination. Whether it's Evelyn's persistence, Harold's slow rebuilding of trust in his body, or Margaret's community of support, each story reminds us that recovery is a team effort—one that requires as much emotional strength as physical effort. With the right mindset and support, every senior can rebuild and recover, no matter how challenging the road may seem.

CHAPTER 8

HOME-BASED REHABILITATION

Rehabilitation after an injury doesn't always have to take place in a clinic or hospital setting. In fact, many seniors find that home-based rehabilitation provides both convenience and comfort. The familiarity of home can make the recovery process more manageable, and with a few adjustments, it's possible to create an environment that supports healing. In this chapter, we will explore how to adapt the home for safety, the kinds of exercises that can be done without special equipment, and how telemedicine is revolutionizing the way seniors access rehabilitation services from home.

Creating a Safe Home Environment for Recovery: Adapting Spaces to Prevent Re-Injury

After an injury, safety becomes a top priority—especially at home, where slips, trips, and falls are common. Many seniors need to modify their living spaces to prevent re-injury and make everyday activities easier to manage. A safe home environment not only aids in physical recovery but also gives seniors and their caregivers peace of mind.

Consider Bob's story. At 78, Bob had undergone knee surgery and was eager to regain his mobility. However, his home was full of potential hazards—loose rugs, cluttered walkways, and narrow doorways. His physical therapist recommended a home safety assessment, which helped him make several small but impactful changes. He removed the rugs, added grab bars in the bathroom, and placed non-slip mats in key areas like the kitchen and shower. Bob's recovery was smoother and quicker because his home supported his needs rather than posing a risk.

For seniors like Bob, small adjustments can make a world of difference. Some key recommendations for creating a safe home environment include:

- Decluttering walkways: Ensure that hallways and frequently used areas are free from obstacles like furniture or cords.
- Installing grab bars: Placing grab bars in the bathroom and near stairs provides added stability.
- Using non-slip mats: Adding non-slip mats in the shower, bathroom, and kitchen can prevent slips on wet surfaces.
- Rearranging furniture: Move commonly used items to easy-to-reach places so there's no need to climb or bend.
- Improving lighting: Bright, well-placed lighting can help seniors avoid trips or falls in dim areas.

These changes might seem simple, but they play a critical role in allowing seniors to focus on their recovery without worrying about accidents. Having a safe space to move freely encourages physical activity, which is essential for rehabilitation.

Exercises You Can Do at Home: Practical Routines That Don't Require Special Equipment

While professional physical therapy sessions are often necessary, many seniors can supplement their recovery with exercises that can be done at home. These routines don't require expensive or specialized equipment, making them accessible to everyone. The key is consistency—doing these exercises regularly helps maintain mobility, strength, and flexibility.

Take Mary's experience. After recovering from a back injury, Mary's physical therapist gave her a series of at-home exercises to continue strengthening her core. She was hesitant at first, unsure if she could stay motivated without someone guiding her. But with a simple routine of seated leg lifts, gentle stretches, and balancing exercises, Mary found she was able to keep progressing. Doing these exercises in the comfort of her living room, she started to regain the strength in her lower back and noticed a significant improvement in her pain levels.

Here are a few practical exercises that can be easily done at home:

- Seated leg lifts: While sitting in a chair, raise one leg at a time, holding it in the air for a few seconds before lowering it. This helps strengthen leg muscles without putting pressure on joints.

- Standing heel raises: Hold onto a chair or counter for balance and slowly rise onto the balls of your feet, then lower yourself back down. This improves calf strength and stability.

- Wall push-ups: Stand facing a wall and place your hands against it at shoulder height. Slowly lower your body toward the wall and then push back. This helps build upper body strength.

- Ankle circles: While seated, lift one foot slightly off the ground and make circles with your ankle. This promotes flexibility and circulation in the lower legs.

- Gentle stretches: Simple stretches for the neck, shoulders, and legs can help maintain flexibility and reduce stiffness.

These exercises are low-impact and can be modified based on each person's mobility and fitness level. Even seniors with limited range of motion or balance issues can benefit from seated or supported variations. The most important thing is to stay active and engaged with the rehabilitation process.

Telemedicine and Virtual Physical Therapy: Accessing Professional Care from Home

In recent years, telemedicine has revolutionized healthcare, and physical therapy is no exception. With virtual consultations, seniors can now receive professional care and guidance without leaving the comfort of their homes. This is particularly beneficial for those who may have limited access to in-person services due to mobility issues or living in rural areas.

Jean, an 82-year-old retiree, found herself needing rehabilitation after a shoulder injury but lived in a small town with limited healthcare services. She was introduced to telemedicine by her doctor, and soon she was attending virtual physical therapy sessions. Using her tablet, Jean followed along with exercises demonstrated by her therapist and received feedback on her form. This remote care allowed Jean to stay consistent with her rehabilitation without the burden of travel or waiting for appointments.

Telemedicine offers numerous benefits for seniors, including:

- Convenience: Sessions can be scheduled around the senior's lifestyle and energy levels, and there's no need to travel to a clinic.

- Access to specialized care: Seniors who live far from urban centers can still access experts who specialize in geriatric rehabilitation.

- Real-time feedback: Virtual sessions allow therapists to watch seniors perform exercises and offer guidance on how to improve their technique.

- Increased independence: Telemedicine empowers seniors to take an active role in their recovery, as they can access care from their own homes.

For those interested in virtual rehabilitation, it's important to have the right setup. A device with a camera and internet access, such as a tablet or computer, is usually necessary. Some therapists may recommend additional equipment, like resistance bands or small weights, but many exercises can be done with household items or body weight.

Virtual physical therapy isn't just a temporary solution; it's becoming an integral part of modern rehabilitation. For seniors who are homebound or prefer the convenience of online sessions, telemedicine bridges the gap, ensuring that they receive the professional care they need without the limitations of location.

Home-based rehabilitation offers seniors the opportunity to recover in a space that's familiar and comfortable. By creating a safe home environment, incorporating simple exercises, and embracing the advantages of telemedicine, seniors can take control of their recovery and achieve their rehabilitation goals. Whether it's Bob's modified living room, Mary's at-home exercise routine, or Jean's virtual therapy sessions, these stories remind us that healing can happen anywhere—with the right support and guidance.

The flexibility of home-based rehabilitation empowers seniors to stay active and engaged in their recovery. With the right adjustments and a commitment to daily practice, seniors can rebuild strength, prevent future injuries, and ultimately regain their independence—all from the comfort of home.

CHAPTER 9

POST-REHABILITATION MAINTENANCE

Completing a rehabilitation program is a major milestone in any senior's recovery journey. But the work doesn't stop once the structured therapy sessions end. In fact, maintaining the gains achieved during rehabilitation is essential for preventing future injuries and staying strong. This chapter explores how seniors can continue to build on their progress, strategies for staying active long-term, and signs that further rehabilitation or medical attention may be necessary.

Preventing Future Injuries: Long-Term Strategies to Stay Strong and Agile

For many seniors, the fear of re-injury can loom large after completing rehabilitation. Whether it was a broken bone, a joint replacement, or a soft tissue injury, the road to recovery can be tough, and the last thing anyone wants is to go through it again. Fortunately, there are ways to reduce the risk of future injuries and promote long-term strength and agility.

Margaret's story is an example of how prevention can become part of daily life. After recovering from a hip fracture, she knew that she had to make lifestyle changes to keep her bones strong and her balance steady. Margaret joined a local fitness group that focused on gentle strength training and balance exercises tailored to older adults. She also worked with her physical therapist to learn specific stretches and movements to maintain flexibility in her hips and lower back. These activities not only helped her stay injury-free but also made her feel more confident in her everyday movements.

For seniors like Margaret, preventing future injuries involves:

- Staying physically active: Regular movement is key to maintaining strength, flexibility, and coordination. Even low-impact activities like walking, swimming, and yoga can make a big difference.
- Incorporating balance training: Balance exercises are essential for preventing falls, one of the most common causes of injury in seniors. Simple routines like standing on one foot or practicing heel-to-toe walking can strengthen stabilizing muscles.
- Maintaining bone health: A diet rich in calcium and vitamin D, combined with weight-bearing exercises, helps keep bones strong and less prone to fractures.
- Wearing proper footwear: Supportive shoes with non-slip soles can reduce the risk of falls, especially on slippery or uneven surfaces.
- Being mindful of surroundings: Simple adjustments like installing grab bars, ensuring adequate lighting, and using non-slip mats can make a home environment safer.

By integrating these strategies into daily life, seniors can reduce the likelihood of injury while maintaining their independence and freedom to move with ease.

Sustaining Gains from Rehab: Continuing Exercises for Strength, Balance, and Mobility

The physical and mental benefits gained from rehabilitation don't have to fade once formal therapy ends. Continuing the exercises learned during rehab can help seniors maintain and even enhance their strength, balance, and mobility. The key is to develop a sustainable routine that fits into everyday life.

After completing rehabilitation for a knee injury, Joe knew he needed to keep up with his exercises to avoid stiffness and maintain his range of motion. At first, he found it hard to stay motivated without the structure of regular physical therapy appointments. However, his therapist encouraged him to incorporate the exercises into his morning routine, turning them into a daily habit. By breaking the exercises into small, manageable segments, Joe was able to sustain his gains without feeling overwhelmed.

For seniors like Joe, the following tips can help maintain progress:

- Stick to a routine: Consistency is vital when it comes to maintaining strength and mobility. Aim to set aside time each day for exercises, even if it's just 15 to 20 minutes.
- Keep it simple: It's not necessary to perform complex or high-intensity workouts. Focus on the exercises that target key areas like core stability, leg strength, and flexibility.

- Use household items for resistance: Everyday objects like water bottles, cans, or resistance bands can be used to perform strength-training exercises at home.

- Listen to your body: Pay attention to any discomfort or pain during exercises. It's important to adjust intensity and movements based on how the body feels to avoid overexertion.

- Track progress: Keeping a journal of daily exercises or achievements can provide a sense of accomplishment and motivation to continue.

By integrating these practices, seniors can continue to benefit from the hard work they've put into rehabilitation. Staying active is not only good for physical health but also boosts mood and confidence, leading to a better quality of life.

When to Seek Additional Care: Recognizing Signs That Indicate Further Rehabilitation Is Needed

While many seniors successfully complete rehabilitation and go on to lead active lives, there are times when additional care may be necessary. Understanding when to seek further medical or therapeutic support is crucial for preventing small issues from becoming larger problems.

Mary's experience highlights the importance of recognizing when it's time to reach out for help. After completing her rehabilitation for a shoulder injury, she felt great for several months. However, as time passed, she noticed increasing stiffness in her shoulder, which began to affect her daily activities. At first, she tried to manage it with at-home stretches, but the discomfort persisted. Instead of waiting for the problem to worsen, Mary contacted her doctor, who recommended a follow-up physical therapy program. The additional rehabilitation helped her regain mobility and prevent long-term issues.

Here are some signs that may indicate further care or rehabilitation is needed:

- Persistent pain: While some soreness is normal after exercise, lingering or sharp pain should not be ignored. It may signal that the injury hasn't fully healed or that additional therapy is needed.
- Decreased mobility: If there's a noticeable decline in range of motion or difficulty performing movements that were previously easy, it may be time to consult a physical therapist.
- Balance problems: New or worsening balance issues can increase the risk of falls and should be addressed through targeted rehabilitation or medical care.
- Recurrent injuries: If the same injury keeps reoccurring, there may be underlying weaknesses or imbalances that require further attention.
- Fatigue during everyday activities: Struggling with daily tasks like walking, climbing stairs, or carrying groceries may indicate a need for ongoing physical support.

By staying attuned to these signs and seeking professional guidance when needed, seniors can catch potential problems early and avoid more serious complications.

Post-rehabilitation maintenance is about more than just staying active—it's about adopting long-term habits that support overall health and well-being. By preventing future injuries, continuing the exercises learned during rehab, and knowing when to seek additional care, seniors can enjoy a higher quality of life and maintain their independence. As Margaret, Joe, and Mary's stories illustrate, recovery doesn't end when rehabilitation stops—it's a continuous journey toward strength, resilience, and vitality. With the right mindset and tools, seniors can rebuild and recover, while also staying prepared for whatever comes next.

CHAPTER 10

ALTERNATIVE THERAPIES AND ADVANCED TREATMENTS

As seniors navigate the journey of rehabilitation, many discover that traditional therapies aren't the only pathways to recovery. In recent years, alternative therapies and advanced treatments have gained popularity for their ability to complement conventional rehabilitation methods. These approaches often focus on enhancing recovery through gentle movements, relaxation techniques, and innovative technologies. In this chapter, we will explore hydrotherapy, electrical stimulation therapy, and practices like yoga and Tai Chi, all of which can play vital roles in the healing process.

Hydrotherapy and Aqua Aerobics: Water-Based Rehabilitation for Gentle Joint Recovery

Water has long been celebrated for its healing properties, and hydrotherapy is one of the most effective methods for seniors recovering from injuries. The buoyancy of water reduces stress on joints and allows for a greater range of motion while minimizing pain. For many, the water feels like a sanctuary where they can move freely without the burden of gravity.

Take the story of Helen, a spirited 72-year-old who fractured her ankle while gardening. After weeks of being immobile, Helen felt both frustrated and anxious about regaining her strength. Her physical therapist recommended hydrotherapy sessions, which quickly became a highlight of her recovery. Floating and moving in the warm water not only eased her pain but also made her feel weightless and liberated. Through aqua aerobics, she engaged in exercises designed to strengthen her ankle and improve her balance, all while having fun. In hydrotherapy, several benefits become apparent:

- Reduced Pain and Swelling: The warmth of the water can help increase blood flow and reduce swelling, promoting faster healing.
- Improved Strength and Flexibility: Water provides natural resistance, enabling gentle strengthening exercises without the risk of injury that may occur on land.
- Enhanced Mobility: The supportive environment of water allows seniors to move more freely, encouraging increased range of motion and confidence in their movements.

Hydrotherapy can be a vital addition to any rehabilitation program, helping seniors like Helen reclaim their mobility in a safe and enjoyable manner.

Electrical Stimulation Therapy: How Technology Can Help Regain Muscle Function

In the age of modern medicine, technology is stepping in to assist rehabilitation in remarkable ways. Electrical stimulation therapy (EST) uses electrical impulses to stimulate muscles, promoting muscle contraction and aiding in recovery. This method has been particularly beneficial for seniors recovering from strokes, surgeries, or long-term immobilization.

Frank, a retired teacher, experienced this first hand after undergoing knee replacement surgery. Despite his commitment to rehabilitation exercises, he struggled to regain strength in his quadriceps. His physical therapist introduced him to electrical stimulation therapy as part of his recovery plan. With electrodes placed on his thigh muscles, Frank felt a gentle pulsing sensation that triggered muscle contractions. Although initially skeptical, he soon noticed a marked improvement in muscle strength and function.

The advantages of electrical stimulation therapy include:

- Faster Muscle Recovery: By promoting muscle activation, EST can accelerate the rehabilitation process, particularly when combined with traditional exercises.
- Pain Reduction: Many patients find that electrical stimulation helps alleviate discomfort, allowing for a more effective rehabilitation experience.
- Enhanced Coordination: As the muscles strengthen, coordination improves, contributing to overall functional recovery.

As Frank's story illustrates, electrical stimulation therapy can serve as a powerful ally in the rehabilitation toolkit, allowing seniors to regain muscle function and confidence in their movements.

Yoga and Tai Chi for Seniors: Gentle, Adaptable Movements to Aid Recovery

Two ancient practices, yoga and Tai Chi, have gained recognition not just for their physical benefits but also for their mental and emotional support during recovery. Both offer low-impact exercises that promote flexibility, balance, and relaxation, making them ideal for seniors.

Take Anna, an active 68-year-old who turned to yoga after her recovery from a shoulder injury. Initially apprehensive about re-engaging in physical activity, she found solace in a gentle yoga class designed for seniors. The instructor emphasized mindful movements, deep breathing, and modifications to accommodate individual abilities. As Anna progressed, she discovered that yoga not only improved her shoulder's mobility but also brought her a sense of calmness and clarity.

Similarly, Tai Chi, often referred to as "meditation in motion," involves slow, flowing movements that enhance balance and coordination. Tom, a 75-year-old who struggled with stability after a fall, began practicing Tai Chi as a way to build strength and regain confidence. Through consistent practice, he learned to focus on his breath and movements, improving his balance and overall well-being.

The benefits of incorporating yoga and Tai Chi into a rehabilitation regimen include:

- Improved Flexibility: Both practices emphasize stretching and range of motion, which can help prevent stiffness in injured areas.
- Enhanced Balance: The slow, deliberate movements promote stability, reducing the risk of future falls.
- Stress Relief: Mindfulness and deep breathing techniques foster relaxation, helping to alleviate anxiety associated with recovery.

For seniors like Anna and Tom, these gentle practices not only aid physical recovery but also provide emotional support during their healing journeys.

As seniors explore alternative therapies and advanced treatments, they open up new pathways to recovery that can enhance their overall rehabilitation experience. Hydrotherapy offers a soothing environment for gentle movement, electrical stimulation therapy harnesses technology to aid muscle recovery, and practices like yoga and Tai Chi provide holistic benefits that address both body and mind.

These approaches complement traditional rehabilitation methods and empower seniors to take an active role in their healing journeys. By embracing alternative therapies, seniors can rebuild and recover with confidence, transforming their experiences into stories of resilience and triumph. As they discover what works best for their bodies and lifestyles, they are not only healing from injuries but also enriching their lives with new skills, communities, and joy.

CONCLUSION

As we reach the end of this journey through injury rehabilitation for seniors, it's essential to reflect on the key themes that have emerged: resilience, empowerment, and the unwavering spirit of those determined to reclaim their lives after an injury. The road to recovery is not just about healing the body; it is also about nurturing the mind and spirit, fostering independence, and embracing a lifestyle that prioritizes health and well-being.

Staying Active for Life

At the heart of long-term health is the commitment to staying active. Throughout this book, we've explored various physical activities tailored for seniors—everything from low-impact exercises to gentle movements like yoga and Tai Chi. The importance of regular movement cannot be overstated; it enhances strength, balance, and flexibility, ultimately reducing the risk of future injuries.

Take the story of Ruth, a vibrant 70-year-old who took up swimming after her rehabilitation. Initially fearful of water, she found her confidence growing with each session. Over time, swimming became not only a source of physical activity but also a social outlet, connecting her with a community of fellow swimmers. Ruth's experience exemplifies the transformative power of remaining active, proving that movement can invigorate life at any age.

Encouraging a lifestyle centered around regular exercise not only enhances physical health but also contributes to mental clarity and emotional resilience. As seniors incorporate movement into their daily routines, they cultivate a sense of purpose and vitality, setting the stage for a more fulfilled life.

Reclaiming Independence

Rehabilitation is a pathway to renewed freedom. It offers seniors the tools to regain their independence, allowing them to navigate their daily lives with confidence. The journey may be challenging, but the rewards are profound.

Consider the journey of James, who, after recovering from a hip fracture, embraced a personalized rehabilitation program that included strength training and balance exercises. With determination and support from his family and therapists, he not only regained his mobility but also returned to activities he loved, like gardening and playing with his grandchildren. James's story is a testament to how rehabilitation can empower individuals to reclaim their independence, transforming their lives and reconnecting them with their passions.

As seniors work through their rehabilitation programs, it's crucial to celebrate milestones, however small they may seem. Each step forward is a victory that brings a sense of achievement and fosters a deeper belief in one's abilities. With newfound independence, seniors can explore life beyond injury, enjoying experiences and adventures they might have thought were lost.

The journey of recovery is often fraught with obstacles, but within each challenge lies the opportunity for growth. Resilience and determination are powerful forces that can guide seniors through even the toughest times.

Whether it's coping with setbacks, managing fears of re-injury, or navigating the emotional landscape of recovery, seniors are reminded that they are not alone. With the support of loved ones, healthcare professionals, and community resources, they can rise above adversity and emerge stronger.

As we conclude this book, let it serve as a roadmap to recovery and independence. Embrace the journey, harness the power of movement, and nurture your spirit. The stories of individuals like Ruth and James remind us that recovery is not just a destination; it is a lifelong journey filled with possibilities, discoveries, and triumphs.

The road may be winding, but every step taken in pursuit of health and independence is a testament to the resilience of the human spirit. As you embark on your rehabilitation journey or support a loved one through theirs, remember that healing is not only about restoring physical strength but also about cultivating a life rich in purpose, connection, and joy. The journey ahead is filled with hope and the promise of renewed freedom—embrace it wholeheartedly.

9 798304 755832